Complete Keto Diet Cookbook

Easy-to-prepare Keto ideas for everyday meals

Kayleigh Lawson

TABLE OF CONTENTS

Readers acknowledge that the author is not engaging in the rendering of legal, financial, medical or professional advice. The content within this book has been derived from various sources. Please consult a licensed professional before attempting any techniques outlined in this book. By reading this document, the reader agrees that under no circumstances is the author responsible for any losses, 5 direct or indirect, which are incurred as a result of the use of information contained within this document, including, but not limited to, — errors, omissions, or inaccuracies.

BREAKFAST

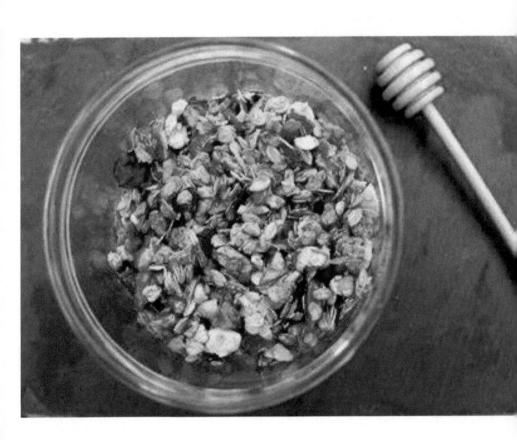

Breakfast Meatloaf

Servings: 4

Cooking Time: 35 minutes

Ingredients

- 1 teaspoon ghee
- 1 small yellow onion, chopped
- 1 pound sweet sausage, chopped
- 6 eggs
- 1 cup cheddar cheese, shredded
- 4 ounces cream cheese, soft
- Salt and black pepper to the taste
- 2 tablespoons scallions, chopped

Directions:

1. Mix eggs with salt, pepper, onion, sausage and half of the cream and whisk well.

2. Grease a meatloaf with the ghee, pour sausage and eggs mix, introduce in the oven at 350 degrees F and bake for minutes.

3. Take the meatloaf out of the oven, leave aside for a couple of minutes, spread the rest of the cream cheese on top and sprinkle scallions and cheddar cheese all over.

4. Introduce meatloaf in the oven again and bake for 5 minutes more.

5. After the time has passed, broil meatloaf for 3 minutes, leave it aside to cool down a bit, slice and serve it.

6. Enjoy!

Nutrition Info:

Calories 560, fat 32, fiber 1, carbs 6, protein 45

Coconut Muesli

Servings: 15

Preparation Time: 1 minute

Cooking Time: 8 minutes

Ingredients:

- Flaked coconut -unsweetened: 1 cup
- Sunflower seeds: 1 cup
- Pumpkin seeds: 1 cup
- Almonds -sliced: 1 cup
- Pecans: ½ cup
- Hemp hearts: ½ cup
- Cinnamon: 2 teaspoons
- Vanilla extract: ½ teaspoon
- Vanilla stevia: ¼ teaspoon

Directions:

1. Toss together all the ingredients in a baking pan.
2. Bake for 7-8 minutes at 350 degrees Fahrenheit.
3. Leave to cool.
4. Serve with almond milk.

Nutrition Value:

200 Cal, 17.8 g total fat, 3 mg sodium, 6.1 g carb., 3.3g fiber, 6.9 g protein.

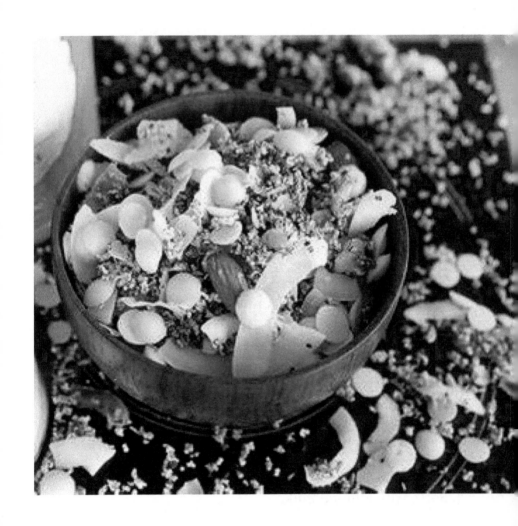

Fruit & Nut Cereal

Servings: 1

Preparation Time: 5 minutes

Ingredients:

- Strawberries -chopped: 2
- Blueberries: 2 tablespoon
- Almonds -chopped: 3 tablespoon
- Walnuts -chopped: 2 tablespoon
- Pecans -chopped: 3 tablespoon
- Sweetener: 3 tablespoon
- Coconut milk: for serving

Directions:

1. Combine together all the ingredients in a bowl except the coconut milk.

2. Stir in the coconut milk.

Nutrition Value:

308 Cal, 32.59 g total fat, 2.96g carb., 5.79g fiber, 7.88 g protein.

Blueberry Porridge

Servings: 2

Preparation Time: 5 minutes

Cooking Time: 5 minutes

Ingredients:

- Almond milk: 1 cup
- Ground flaxseed: ¼ cup
- Coconut flour: ¼ cup
- Cinnamon: 1 teaspoon
- Vanilla extract: 1 teaspoon
- Liquid stevia: 10 drops
- Salt: a pinch

Directions:

1. Heat the almond milk over a low flame and whisk in the flour, flaxseed, salt, and cinnamon.
2. Mix in the vanilla extract and stevia once it begins to bubble.
3. Remove from the flame once the mixture is thick.
4. Serve topped with shaved coconut, pumpkin seeds, and some blueberries.

Nutrition Value:

405 Cal, 34 g total fat, 8 g net carb., 10 g protein.

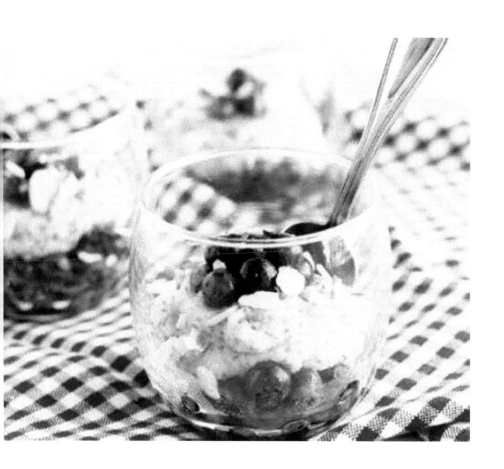

Morning Berry-green Smoothie

Servings: 4

Cooking Time: 5 minutes

Ingredients

- 1 avocado, pitted and sliced
- 3 cups mixed blueberries and strawberries
- 2 cups unsweetened almond milk
- 6 tbsp heavy cream
- 2 tbsp erythritol
- 1 cup of ice cubes
- ⅓ cup nuts and seeds mix

Directions:

1. Combine the avocado slices, blueberries, strawberries, almond milk, heavy cream, erythritol, ice cubes, nuts and seeds in a smoothie maker; blend at high speed until smooth and uniform.

2. Pour the smoothie into drinking glasses and serve immediately.

Nutrition Info (Per Serving): Kcal 360, Fat 33.3g, Net Carbs 6g, Protein 6g

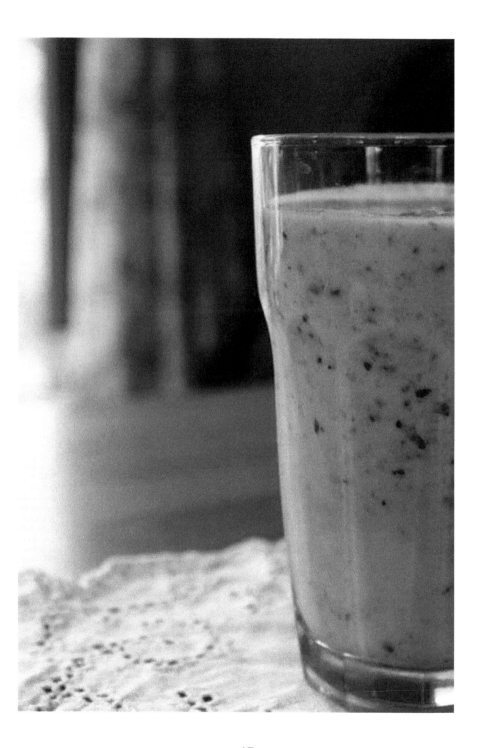

BRUNCH

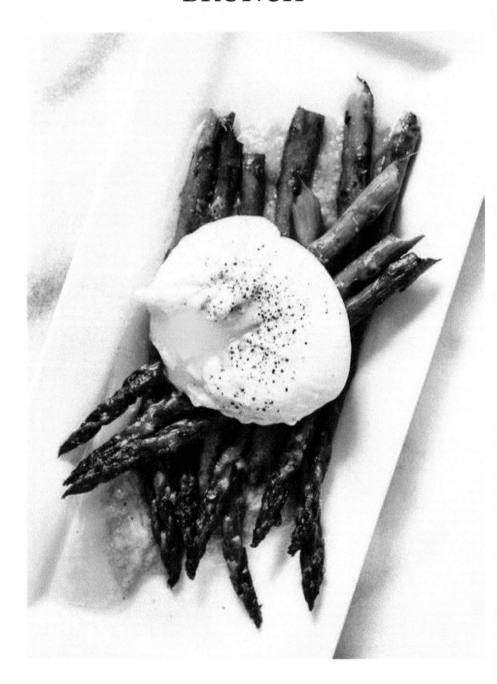

Avocado Halloumi Scones

Servings: 4

Cooking Time: 35 minutes

Ingredients

- 1 cup crumbled halloumi cheese
- 2 cups almond flour
- 3 tsp baking powder
- ½ cup butter, cold
- 1 avocado, pitted and mashed
- 1 large egg
- 1/3 cup buttermilk

Directions:

1. Preheat oven to 350° F; then line a baking sheet with parchment paper. In a bowl, combine flour and baking powder.

2. Add butter and mix. Top with halloumi cheese, avocado, and combine again.

3. Whisk the egg with the buttermilk and stir in the halloumi mix. Mold 8- scones out to the batter.

4. Place on the baking sheet, then bakes for 25 minutes or until the scones turn a golden color.

5. Let cool.

Nutrition Info (Per Serving): Cal 432; Net Carbs 2.3g; Fat 42g; Protein 10g

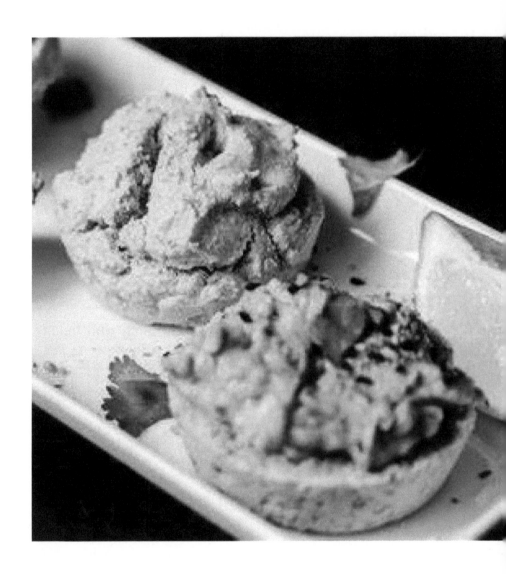

Lunch Spinach Rolls

Servings: 16

Cooking Time: 15 minutes

Ingredients

- 6 tablespoons coconut flour
- ½ cup almond flour
- 2 and ½ cups mozzarella cheese, shredded
- 2 eggs
- A pinch of salt

For the filling:

- 4 ounces cream cheese
- 6 ounces spinach, torn
- A drizzle of avocado oil
- A pinch of salt
- ¼ cup parmesan, grated
- Mayonnaise for serving

Directions:

1. Heat up a pan. Oil over medium heat, add some spinach and cook for 2 minutes.
2. Add parmesan, a pinch of salt and cream cheese, stir well, take off the heat and leave aside for now.

3. Put mozzarella cheese in a heatproof bowl and microwave for seconds.

4. Add eggs, salt, coconut and almond flour and stir everything.

5. Place dough on a lined cutting board, place parchment paper on top and flatten dough with a rolling pin.

6. Divide dough into 1rectangles, spread spinach mix on each and roll them into cigar shapes.

7. Place all rolls on a lined baking sheet, introduce in the oven at 350 degrees F and bake for 15 minutes.

8. Leave rolls to cool down for a few minutes before serving them with some mayo on top.

9. Enjoy!

Nutrition Info: calories 500, fat 65, fiber 4, carbs 14, protein 32

Herbed Coconut Flour Bread

Servings: 2

Cooking Time: 3 minutes

Ingredients

- 4 tbsp coconut flour
- ½ tsp baking powder
- ½ tsp dried thyme
- 2 tbsp whipping cream
- 2 eggs

Seasoning:

- ½ tsp oregano
- 2 tbsp avocado oil

Directions:

1. Take a medium bowl, place all the ingredients in it and then whisk until incorporated and smooth batter comes together.

2. Distribute the mixture evenly between two mugs and then microwave for a minute and 30 seconds until cooked. When done, take out bread from the mugs, cut it into slices, and then serve.

Nutrition Info:

309 Calories; 26.1 g Fats; 9.3 g Protein; 4.3 g Net Carb; 5 g Fiber

Simple Asparagus Lunch

Servings: 4

Cooking Time: 10 minutes

Ingredients

- 2 egg yolks
- Salt and black pepper to the taste
- ¼ cup ghee
- 1 tablespoon lemon juice
- A pinch of cayenne pepper
- 40 asparagus spears

Directions:

1. In a bowl, whisk egg yolks very well.
2. Transfer this to a small pan over low heat.
3. Add lemon juice and whisk well.
4. Add ghee and whisk until it melts.
5. Add salt, pepper, cayenne pepper and whisk again well.
6. Heat up a pan at medium-high heat, add asparagus spears and fry them for 5 minutes.
7. Divide asparagus between plates, drizzle the sauce you've made on top and serve.
8. Enjoy!

Nutrition Info: calories 150, fat 13, fiber 6, carbs 2, protein 3

Herbed Keto Bread

Servings: 6

Cooking Time: 40 minutes

Ingredients

- 5 eggs
- ½ tsp cream of tartar
- 2 cups almond flour
- 3 tablespoons butter, melted
- 3 tsp baking powder
- 1 tsp salt
- 1 tsp dried rosemary
- ½ tsp dried oregano
- 1 tbsp sunflower seeds
- 2 tbsp sesame seeds

Directions:

1. Preheat oven to 360° F, then grease a loaf pan with cooking spray. Combine the eggs with cream of tartar until the formation of stiff peaks happens. In a food processor, place in the baking powder, flour, salt, and butter and blitz to incorporate fully.

2. Stir in the egg mixture. Ladle the batter into the prepared loaf pan. Spread the loaf with sesame seeds, dried rosemary, sunflower seeds, and oregano and bake for 35 minutes. Serve with butter.

Nutrition Info (Per Serving):

Kcal 115, Fat: 10.2g, Net Carbs: 1g, Protein: 3.9g

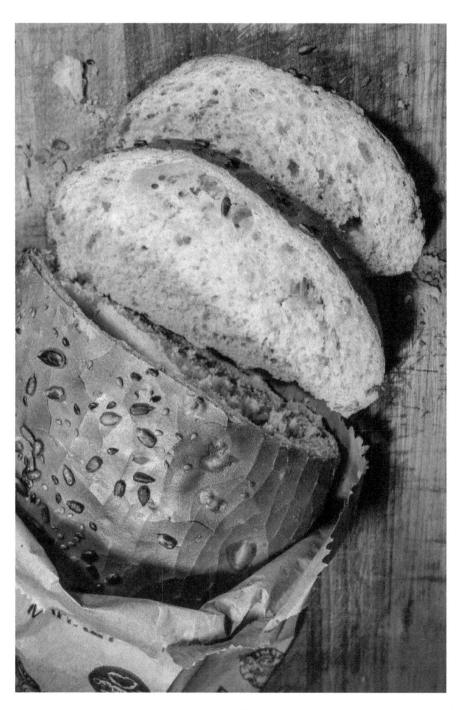

SOUP AND STEWS

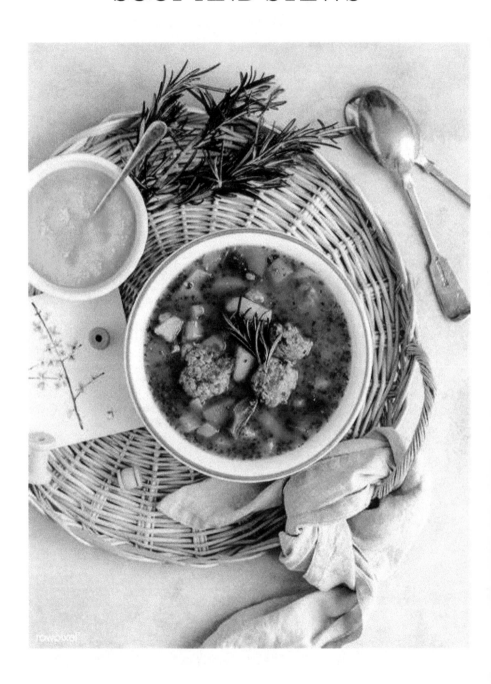

Mixed Mushroom Soup

Servings: 4

Cooking Time: 35 minutes

Ingredients

- 5 oz white button mushrooms, chopped
- 5 oz cremini mushrooms, chopped
- 5 oz shiitake mushrooms, chopped
- 4 oz unsalted butter
- 1 small onion, finely chopped
- 1 clove garlic, minced
- ½ lb celery root, chopped
- ½ tsp dried rosemary
- 4 cups of water
- 1 vegan stock cube, crushed
- 1 tbsp plain vinegar
- 1 cup coconut cream
- 6 leaves basil, chopped

Directions:

1. Melt butter in a saucepan. Sauté onion, garlic, mushrooms, and celery root until golden brown and fragrant, about 6 minutes.
2. Reserve some mushrooms for garnishing. Add in rosemary, water, stock cube, and vinegar.

3. Stir and bring to a boil for 6 minutes.

4. Reduce the heat and simmer for minutes.

5. Mix in coconut cream and puree.

6. Spoon into bowls garnished with the reserved mushrooms and basil.

Nutrition Info (Per Serving):

Cal 506; Fat 46g; Net Carbs 12g; Protein 8g

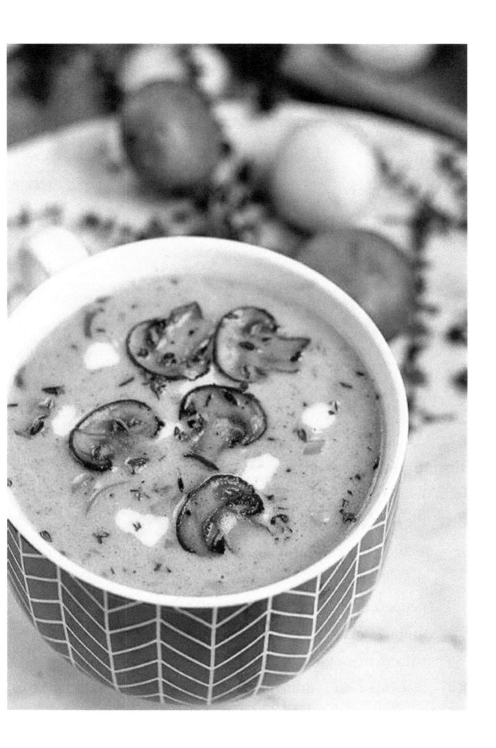

Creamy Cauliflower Soup with Bacon Chips

Servings: 4

Cooking Time: 25 minutes

Ingredients

- 2 tbsp ghee
- 1 onion, chopped
- 2 head cauliflower, cut into florets
- 2 cups of water
- Salt and black pepper to taste
- 3 cups almond milk
- 1 cup shredded white cheddar cheese
- 3 bacon strips

Directions:

1. Melt the ghee into a saucepan, over medium heat and sauté the onion for 3 minutes until fragrant.

2. Include the cauli florets, sauté for 3 minutes to slightly soften, add the water, and season with salt and black pepper. Bring to a boil; then, you need to reduce the heat to low. Cover and cook for 10 minutes. Puree cauliflower with an immersion blender until the ingredients are evenly combined, and stir in the almond milk and cheese until the cheese melts. Adjust taste with salt and black pepper.

3. In a non-stick skillet over high heat, fry the bacon until crispy. Divide soup between serving bowls, top with crispy bacon, and serve hot.

Nutrition Info (Per Serving): Kcal 402, Fat 37g, Net Carbs 6g, Protein 8g

Roasted Tomato Cream

Servings: 8

Cooking Time: 1 Hour

Ingredients

- 1 jalapeno pepper, chopped
- 4 garlic cloves, minced
- 2 pounds cherry tomatoes, cut in halves
- 1 yellow onion, cut into wedges
- Salt and black pepper to the taste
- ¼ cup olive oil
- ½ teaspoon oregano, dried
- 4 cups chicken stock
- ¼ cup basil, chopped
- ½ cup parmesan, grated

Directions:

1. Spread tomatoes and onion in a baking dish. Add garlic and chili pepper, season with salt, pepper and oregano and drizzle the oil.

2. Toss to coat and bake in the oven at 4 degrees F for 30 minutes.

3. Take tomatoes to mix out of the oven, transfer to a pot, add stock and heat everything up over medium-high heat.

4. Bring to a boil, cover the pot, reduce heat and simmer for 20 minutes.

5. Blend using an immersion blender, add salt and pepper to the taste and basil, stir and ladle into soup bowls.

6. Sprinkle parmesan on top and serve.

7. Enjoy!

Nutrition Info: calories 140, fat 2, fiber 2, carbs 5, protein 8

Nutmeg Pumpkin Soup

Preparation Time: 15 minutes

Cooking Time: 20 minutes

Servings: 4

Ingredients:

- 1 tablespoon of butter
- 1 onion (diced)
- 1 16-ounce can of pumpkin puree
- 1 1/3 cups of vegetable broth
- 1/2 tablespoon of nutmeg
- 1/2 tablespoon of sugar Salt (to taste)
- Pepper (to taste)
- 3 cups of soymilk or any milk as a substitute

Directions:

1. Using a large saucepan, add onion to margarine and cook it between 3 and 5 minutes until the onion is clear
2. Add pumpkin puree, vegetable broth, sugar, pepper, and other ingredients and stir to combine.
3. Cook in medium heat for between 10 and fifteen minutes
4. Before serving the soup, taste and add more spices, pepper, and salt if necessary. Serve soup and enjoy it!

Nutrition:

Calories: 165 Fat: 4.9g Fiber: 11.9g Carbohydrates: 3.5 g Protein: 4.2g

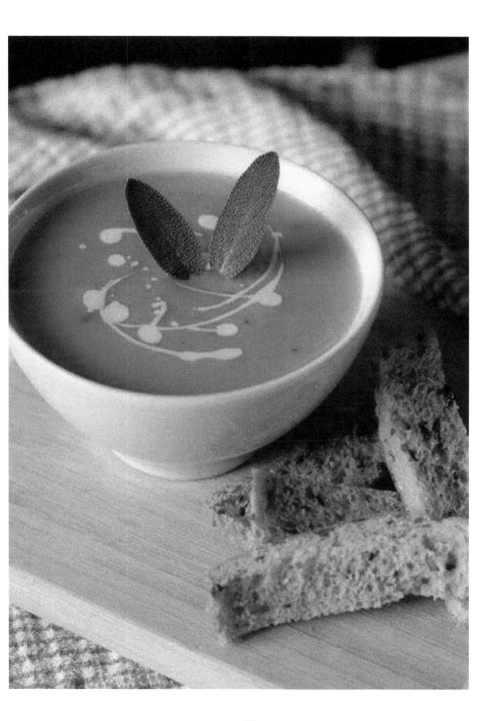

Thai Coconut Vegetable Soup

Preparation Time: 15 minutes

Cooking Time: 20 minutes

Servings: 4

Ingredients:

- onion (diced)
- bell peppers (red, diced)
- 1/4 teaspoon of cayenne
- 1/2 tablespoon of coriander
- 1/2 tablespoon of cumin
- 4 tablespoons of olive oil
- 1 can of chickpeas
- 1 carrot (sliced)
- 3 cloves of garlic
- 1/2 cup of basil or cilantro (fresh chopped)
- 1 teaspoon of salt
- 3 limes (freshly squeezed juice)
- 1/2 cup of vegetable broth
- 1 cup of coconut milk
- 1 cup of peanut butter
- 21/2 cups of tomatoes (finely diced)

Directions:

1. Sauté garlic and onions. Make ingredients to be soft for at least 3 to 5 minutes

2. Leaving out basil, add the rest of the ingredients and allow it to simmer. Cook over low heat for an hour

3. Put the half amount to the food processor, allow it to be very smooth, and return to the pot

4. Add either basil or cilantro, and your coconut food is ready. Before serving the soup, taste and add more seasoning if necessary. Serve, and enjoy!

Nutrition:

Calories: 151 Fat: 6.9g Fiber: 12.5g Carbohydrates: 3.1 g Protein: 4.9g

MAIN

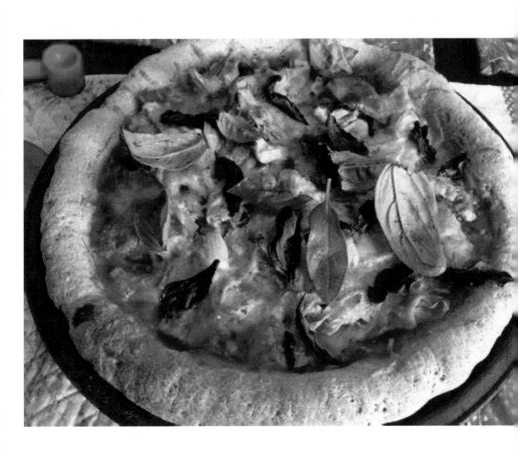

Cheesy Bacon Squash Spaghetti

Preparation Time: 30 minutes

Cooking Time: 50 minutes

Servings: 4

Ingredients:

- 2 pounds spaghetti squash
- 2 pounds bacon
- 1/2 cup of butter
- 2 cups of shredded parmesan cheese
- Salt
- Black pepper

Directions:

1. Let the oven preheat to 375° F.

2. Trim or remove each spaghetti squash stem, slice into rings no more than an inch wide, and take out the seeds.

3. Lay the sliced rings down on the baking sheet, bake for 40-45 minutes.

4. It is ready when the strands separate easily when a fork is used to scrape it. Let it cool.

5. Cook sliced up bacon until crispy. Take out and let it cool.

6. Take off the shell on each ring, separate each strand with a fork, and put them in a bowl.

7. Heat the strands in a microwave to get them warm, put in butter, and stir around until the butter melts.

8. Pour in parmesan cheese and bacon crumbles, and add salt and pepper to your taste.

9. Enjoy.

Nutrition:

Calories: 398 Fat: 12.5g Fiber: 9.4g Carbohydrates: 4.1 g Protein: 5.1g

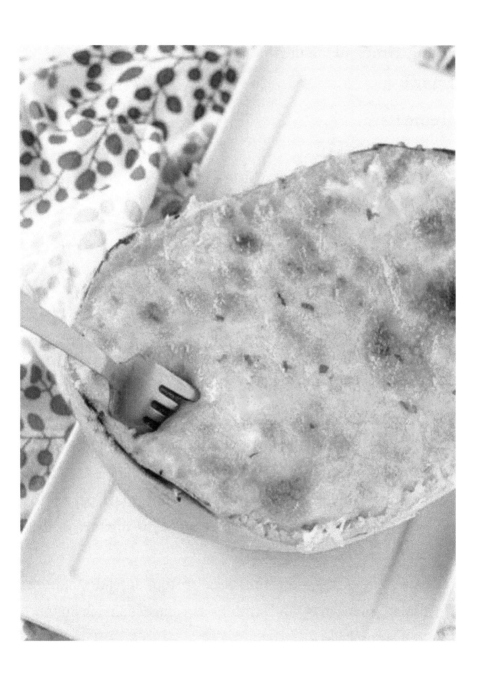

Spinach and Zucchini Lasagna

Preparation Time: 15 minutes

Cooking Time: 30 minutes

Servings: 4

Ingredients:

- zucchinis, sliced
- Salt and black pepper to taste
- 2 cups ricotta cheese
- 2 cups shredded mozzarella cheese
- 3 cups tomato sauce
- 1 cup baby spinach

Directions:

1. Let the oven heat to 375 and grease a baking dish with cooking spray. Put the zucchini slices in a colander and sprinkle with salt.

2. Let sit and drain liquid for 5 minutes and pat dry with paper towels.

3. Mix the ricotta, mozzarella cheese, salt, and black pepper to evenly combine and spread 1/4 cup of the mixture in the bottom of the baking dish.

4. Layer 1/3 of the zucchini slices on top, spread 1 cup of tomato sauce over, and scatter a 1/3 cup of spinach on top. Repeat process.

5. Grease one end of foil with cooking spray and cover the baking dish with the foil.

6. Let it bake for about 35 minutes. And bake further for 5 to 10 minutes or until the cheese has a nice golden-brown color.

7. Remove the dish, sit for 5 minutes, make slices of the lasagna, and serve warm.

Nutrition:

Calories: 376 Fat: 14.1g Fiber: 11.3g Carbohydrates: 2.1 g Protein: 9.5g

Tomato Artichoke Pizza

Servings: 4

Cooking Time: 40 minutes

Ingredients

- 2 oz canned artichokes, cut into wedges
- 2 tbsp flax seed powder
- 4¼ oz grated broccoli
- 6¼ oz grated Parmesan
- ½ tsp salt
- 2 tbsp tomato sauce
- 2 oz mozzarella cheese, grated
- 1 garlic clove, thinly sliced
- 1 tbsp dried oregano
- Green olives for garnish

Directions:

1. Preheat oven to 350° F, then line a baking sheet with parchment paper.
2. In a bowl, mix flax seed powder and 6 tbsp water and allow thickening for 5 minutes.
3. When the flax egg is ready, add broccoli, 4 ½ ounces of Parmesan cheese, salt, and stir to combine.
4. Pour the mixture into the baking sheet and bake until the crust is lightly browned, 20 minutes. Remove from oven

and spread tomato sauce on top, sprinkle with the remaining Parmesan and mozzarella cheeses, add artichokes and garlic. Spread oregano on top.

5. Bake pizza for minutes at 420° F. Garnish with olives.

Nutrition Info (Per Serving): Cal 860; Net Carbs 10g; Fat 63g; Protein 55g

Cauliflower Risotto with Mushrooms

Servings: 4

Cooking Time: 15 minutes

Ingredients

- 2 shallots, diced
- 3 tbsp olive oil
- ¼ cup veggie broth
- ⅓ cup Parmesan cheese, shredded
- 2 tbsp butter
- 3 tbsp chopped chives
- 2 pounds mushrooms, sliced
- 4 cups cauliflower rice
- Salt and black pepper to taste
- 2 tbsp parsley, chopped

Directions:

1. Heat olive oil in a saucepan over medium heat. Add the mushrooms and shallots and cook for about 5 minutes until tender. Remove from the pan and set aside.

2. Add in the cauliflower, broth, salt, and black pepper, and cook until the liquid is absorbed about 4-5 minutes. Stir in butter and Parmesan cheese until the cheese is melted. Sprinkle with parsley to serve.

Nutrition Info (Per Serving):

Kcal 264, Fat: 18g, Net Carbs: 8.4g

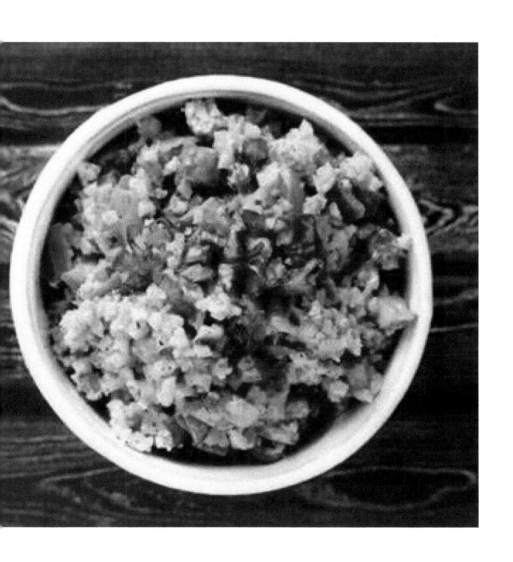

MEAT

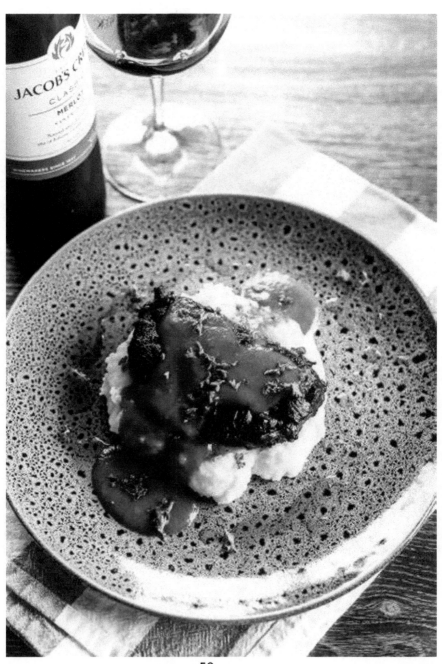

Kalua Pork with Cabbage

Preparation Time: 10 minutes

Cooking Time: 8 hrs.

Servings: 4

Ingredients:

- 1-pound boneless pork butt roast
- Pink Himalayan salt
- Freshly ground black pepper
- tablespoon smoked paprika or Liquid Smoke
- 1/2 cup of water
- 1/2 head cabbage, chopped

Directions:

1. With the crock insert in place, preheat the slow cooker to low.

2. Generously season the pork roast with pink Himalayan salt, pepper, and smoked paprika.

3. Place the pork roast in the slow-cooker insert, and add the water. Cover and cook on low for 7 hours.

4. Transfer the cooked pork roast to a plate. Put the chopped cabbage in the bottom of the slow cooker, and put the pork roast back in on the cabbage. Cover and cook the cabbage and pork roast for 1 hour.

5. Remove the pork roast from the slow cooker and place it on a baking sheet. Use two forks to shred the pork.

6. Serve the shredded pork hot with the cooked cabbage.

7. Reserve the liquid from the slow cooker to remoisten the pork and cabbage when reheating leftovers.

Nutrition:

Calories: 451 Fat: 19.3g Fiber: 11.2g Carbohydrates: 2.1 g Protein: 14.3g

Pork Chops in Blue Cheese Sauce

Preparation Time: 5 minutes

Cooking Time: 10 minutes

Servings: 2

Ingredients:

- boneless pork chops
- Pink Himalayan salt
- Freshly ground black pepper
- 2 tablespoons butter
- 1/3 cup blue cheese crumbles
- 1/3 cup heavy (whipping) cream
- 1/3 cup sour cream

Directions:

1. Dry the pork chops and season with pink Himalayan salt and pepper.

2. In a medium skillet over medium heat, melt the butter. When the butter melts and is very hot, add the pork chops and sear on each side for 3 minutes.

3. The pork chops must be transferred to a plate and let rest for 3 to 5 minutes.

4. In a preheated pan, melt the blue cheese crumbles, frequently stirring, so they don't burn.

5. Add the cream and the sour cream to the pan with the blue cheese. Let simmer for a few minutes, stirring occasionally.

6. For an extra kick of flavor in the sauce, pour the pork-chop pan juice into the cheese mixture and stir. Let simmer while the pork chops are resting.

7. Put the pork chops on two plates, pour the blue cheese sauce over each other, and serve.

Nutrition:

Calories: 434 Fat: 14.1g Fiber: 11.3g Carbohydrates: 3.1 g Protein: 17.5g

Beef and Vegetable Skillet

Preparation Time: 5 minutes

Cooking Time: 15 minutes

Servings: 2

Ingredients:

- 3 oz spinach, chopped
- 1/2 pound ground beef
- 2 slices of bacon, diced
- 2 oz chopped asparagus

Seasoning:

- 3 tbsp. coconut oil
- 2 tsp. dried thyme
- 2/3 tsp. salt
- 1/2 tsp. ground black pepper

Directions:

1. Take a skillet pan, place it over medium heat, add oil and when hot, add beef and bacon and cook for 5 to 7 minutes until slightly browned.

2. Then add asparagus and spinach, sprinkle with thyme, stir well and cook for 7 to 10 minutes until thoroughly cooked.

3. Season skillet with salt and black pepper and serve.

Nutrition:

Calories: 332 Fat: 18.4g Fiber: 9.4g Carbohydrates: 3.8 g Protein: 14.1g

Beef Taco Salad

Preparation Time: 10 minutes

Cooking Time: 10 minutes

Servings: 2

Ingredients:

- 1-pound ground beef (80/20)
- 1/4 teaspoon pink Himalayan sea salt
- 1/4 teaspoon freshly ground black pepper
- 1/4 cup mayonnaise
- 2 tablespoons sugar-free ketchup
- 2 tablespoons yellow mustard
- 1 tablespoon dill relish
- (8-ounce) bag shredded lettuce
- 1/2 cup sliced red onion
- 1/2 cup chopped ripe tomato
- 1 dill pickle, sliced
- 1/4 cup shredded cheddar cheese

Directions:

1. In a medium sauté pan or skillet, brown the ground beef, stirring, for 7 to 10 minutes. Season with salt and pepper, then drain the meat, if desired. In a small bowl, combine the mayonnaise, ketchup, mustard, and relish.

2. Fill a large bowl with the shredded lettuce. Top with the beef, red onion, tomato, dill pickle, and cheese. Put dressing, serve.

Nutrition:

Calories: 398 Fat: 15.1g Fiber: 12.9g Carbohydrates: 3.1 g Protein: 14.8g

Delicious Sausage Salad

Servings: 4

Cooking Time: 7 minutes

Ingredients

- 8 pork sausage links, sliced
- 1 pound mixed cherry tomatoes, cut in halves
- 4 cups baby spinach
- 1 tablespoon avocado oil
- 1 pound mozzarella cheese, cubed
- 2 tablespoons lemon juice
- 2/3 cup basil pesto
- Salt and black pepper to the taste

Directions:

1. Heat up a pan with the oil over medium-high heat, add sausage slices, stir and cook them for 4 minutes on each side.
2. Meanwhile, in a salad bowl, mix spinach with mozzarella, tomatoes, salt, pepper, lemon juice, pesto, and toss to coat.
3. Add sausage pieces, toss again and serve.
4. Enjoy!

Nutrition Info: calories 250, fat 12, fiber 3, carbs 8, protein 18

Beef Shanks Braised in Red Wine Sauce

Preparation Time: 20 minutes

Cooking Time: 8 hrs.

Servings: 6

Ingredients:

- 2 tablespoons olive oil
- pounds (907 g) beef shanks
- 2 cups dry red wine
- cups beef stock
- 1 sprig of fresh rosemary
- 5 garlic cloves, finely chopped
- 1 onion, finely chopped
- Pepper and salt

Directions:

1. Heat olive oil.
2. Put the beef shanks into the skillet and fry for 5 to 10 minutes until well browned.
3. The beef shanks halfway through. Set aside.
4. The red wine must be poured into the pot and let simmer.

5. Add the cooked beef shanks, dry red wine, beef stock, rosemary, garlic, onion, salt, and black pepper to the slow cooker. Stir to mix well.

6. Slow cook with the lid on for 8 hrs.

Nutrition:

Calories: 341 Fat: 19.6g Fiber: 10 g Carbohydrates:15.4 g Protein: 21.6g

Herbed Grilled Lamb

Preparation Time: 15 minutes

Cooking Time: 20 minutes

Servings: 6

Ingredients:

- 2 pounds of lamb
- 5 spoons of ghee butter
- 3 tablespoons of Keto mustard
- 2 minced garlic cloves
- 1 1/2 tablespoon of chopped basil
- 1/2 tablespoon of pepper
- 3 tablespoons of olive oil
- 1/2 teaspoon of salt

Directions:

1. Mix butter, mustard, and basil with a pinch of salt to taste. Then, set aside.
2. Mix garlic, salt, and pepper together. Then, add a teaspoon of oil. Season the lamb generously with this mix.
3. Grill the lamb on medium heat until fully cooked.
4. Take butter mix and spread generously on chops and serve hot.

Nutrition:

Calories: 390 Fat: 19.5 g Fiber: 5.9g Carbohydrates: 3.2 g Protein:
18.6 g

Coconut and Lime Steak

Preparation Time: 25 minutes

Cooking Time: 15 minutes

Servings: 4

Ingredients:

- 2 pounds steak, grass-fed
- 1 tablespoon minced garlic
- 1 lime, zested
- 1 teaspoon ginger, grated
- 3/4 teaspoon sea salt
- 1 teaspoon red pepper flakes
- 2 tablespoons lime juice
- 1/2 cup coconut oil, melted

Directions:

1. Take a large bowl and add garlic, ginger, salt, red pepper flakes, lime juice, zest, pour in oil, and whisk until combined.
2. Add the steaks, toss until well coated, and marinate at room temperature for 20 minutes.
3. After 20 minutes, take a large skillet pan, place it over medium-high heat, and when hot, add steaks (cut steaks in half if they don't fit into the pan).
4. Cook the steaks and then transfer them to a cutting board.

5. Let steaks cool for 5 minutes, then slice across the grain and serve.

Nutrition:

Calories: 512 Fat: 17.9g Fiber: 12.5g Carbohydrates: 4.9 g Protein: 19.9g

POULTRY

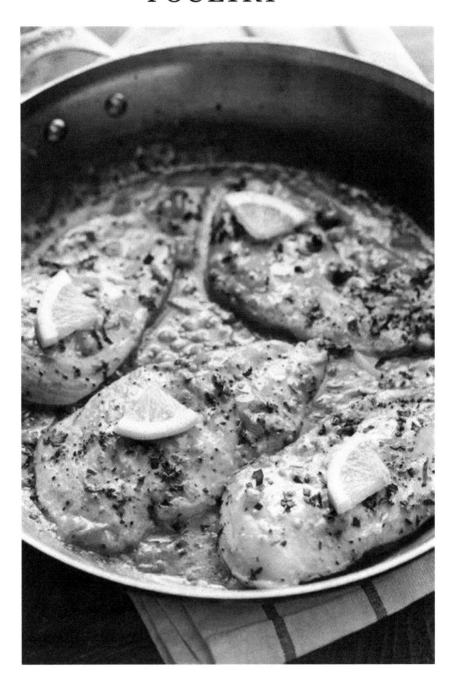

Almond Crusted Chicken Zucchini Stacks

Servings: 4

Cooking Time: 30 minutes

Ingredients

- 1 ½ lb chicken thighs, skinless and boneless, cut into strips
- 3 tbsp almond flour
- Salt and black pepper to taste
- 2 large zucchinis, sliced
- 4 tbsp olive oil
- 2 tsp Italian mixed herb blend
- ½ cup chicken broth

Directions:

1. Preheat oven to 400° F. In a zipper bag, add almond flour, salt, and pepper. Mix and add the chicken slices. Seal the bag and shake to coat.

2. Arrange the zucchinis on a greased baking sheet.

3. Season with salt and pepper, and drizzle with 2 tbsp of olive oil. Remove the chicken from the almond flour mixture, shake off, and put 2-3 chicken strips on each zucchini. Season with an herb blend and drizzle again with olive oil. Bake for 8 minutes; remove the sheet and pour in broth. Bake further for minutes. Serve warm.

Nutrition Info (Per Serving): Cal 512; Net Carbs 1.2g; Fat 42g; Protein 29g

So Delicious Chicken Wings

Servings: 4

Cooking Time: 55 minutes

Ingredients

- 3 pounds of chicken wings
- Salt and black pepper to the taste
- 3 tablespoons coconut aminos
- 2 teaspoons white vinegar
- 3 tablespoons rice vinegar
- 3 tablespoons stevia
- ¼ cup scallions, chopped
- ½ teaspoon xantham gum
- 5 dried chilies, chopped

Directions:

1. Spread chicken wings on a lined baking sheet, season with salt and pepper, introduce in the oven at 375 degrees F and bake for 45 minutes.

2. Meanwhile, heat up a small pan over medium heat, add white vinegar, rice vinegar, coconut aminos, stevia, xantham gum, scallions and chilies, stir well, bring to a boil, cook for minutes and take off the heat.

3. Dip chicken wings into this sauce, arrange them all on the baking sheet again and bake for 10 minutes more.

4. Serve them hot.

5. Enjoy!

Nutrition Info: calories 415, fat 23, fiber 3, carbs 2, protein 27

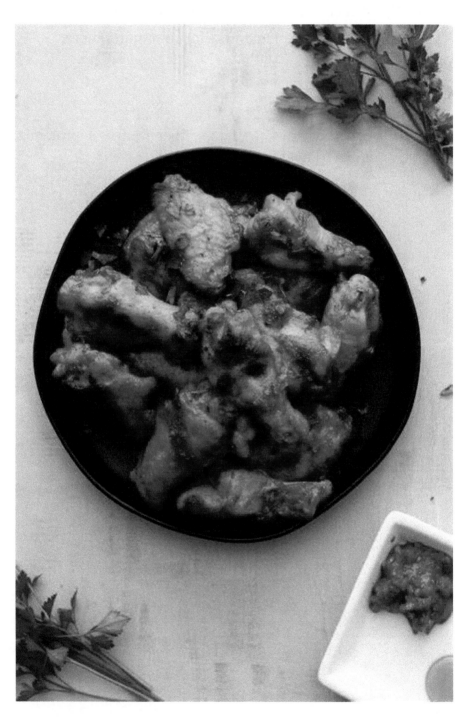

Chicken and Mushrooms

Servings: 4

Cooking Time: 30 minutes

Ingredients

- 1 pound chicken breast, skinless, boneless and cubed
- 2 cups baby bella mushrooms, sliced
- 2 tablespoons olive oil
- 1 red onion, chopped
- 1 red bell pepper, chopped
- 2 garlic cloves, minced
- A pinch of salt and black pepper
- ½ cup chicken stock
- 1 tablespoon balsamic vinegar
- 1 tablespoon parsley, chopped

Directions:

1. Heat up a pan with the oil over medium heat, add the onion and the mushrooms, stir and cook for 5 minutes.

2. Add the chicken, toss and brown for 5 minutes more.

3. Add the rest of the ingredients, toss, bring to a simmer and cook over medium heat for 20 minutes.

4. Divide everything between plates and serve.

Nutrition Info: calories 340, fat 33, fiber 3, carbs 4, protein 20

Creamy Chicken Thighs with Capers

Servings: 4

Cooking Time: 30 minutes

Ingredients

- 2 tbsp butter
- 1 ½ lb chicken thighs
- 2 cups crème fraîche
- 8 oz cream cheese
- 1/3 cup capers
- 1 tbsp tamari sauce

Directions:

1. Heat oven to 350° F and grease a baking sheet. Melt butter in a skillet, season the chicken with salt and pepper and fry until golden brown, 8 minutes.

2. Transfer chicken to the baking sheet, cover with aluminum foil and bake for 8 minutes. Reserve the butter used to sear the chicken.

3. Remove chicken from the oven, take off the foil, and pour the drippings into a pan along with the butter from frying. Set the chicken aside in a warmer for Serves. Place the saucepan over low heat and mix in crème Fraiche and cream cheese.

4. Simmer until the sauce thickens.

5. Mix in capers and tamari sauce; cook further for a minute, and season with salt and pepper. Dish the chicken into plates and drizzle the sauce all over. Serve with buttered broccoli.

Nutrition Info (Per Serving):

Cal 834; Net Carbs 0.9g; Fat 73g; Protein 36g

FISH

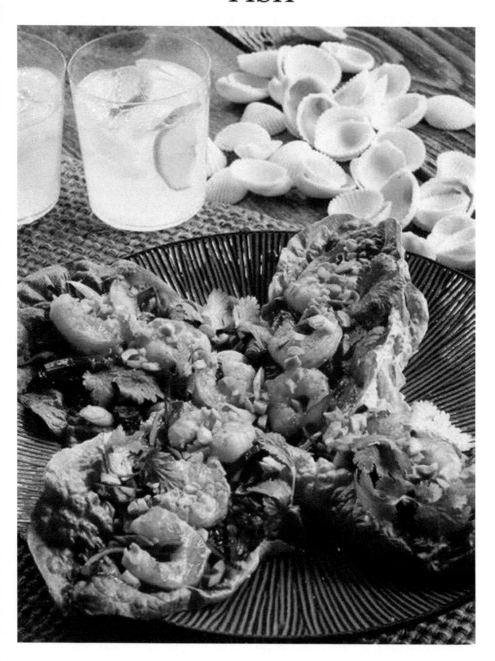

Pistachio-crusted Salmon

Servings: 4

Cooking Time: 35 minutes

Ingredients

- 4 salmon fillets
- ½ tsp pepper
- 1 tsp salt
- ¼ cup mayonnaise
- ½ cup chopped pistachios

Sauce:
- 1 chopped shallot
- 2 tsp lemon zest
- 1 tbsp olive oil
- A pinch of black pepper
- 1 cup heavy cream

Directions:

1. Preheat the oven to 370° F.
2. Brush the salmon with mayonnaise and season with salt and pepper. Coat with pistachios, place in a lined baking dish and bake for 15 minutes.

3. Heat olive oil in a saucepan and sauté the shallot for minutes. Stir in the rest of the sauce ingredients. Bring the mixture to a boil and cook until thickened. Serve the fish with the sauce.

Nutrition Info (Per Serving): Kcal 563, Fat: 47g, Net Carbs: 6g, Protein: 34g

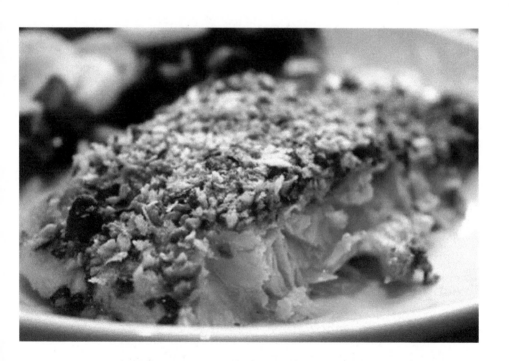

Cod Fillets with Tangy Sesame Sauce

Servings: 6

Cooking Time: 15 minutes

Ingredients

- 6 cod fillets, skin-on
- 3 tablespoons olive oil
- Sea salt and ground black pepper, to season
- 1 lemon, freshly squeezed
- 1/2 teaspoon fresh ginger, minced
- 1 garlic clove, minced
- 1 red chili pepper, minced
- 3 tablespoons toasted sesame seeds
- 3 tablespoons toasted sesame oil

Directions:

1. Prepare a grill for medium-high heat. Rub the cod fillets with olive oil; season both sides with salt and black pepper.

2. Next, place the cod fillets on the grill skin side down. Grill approximately 7 minutes until the skin is lightly charred.

3. To make the sauce, whisk the remaining ingredients until well combined; season with lots of black pepper.

4. Divide the cod fillets among serving plates. Spoon the sauce over them and enjoy!

Nutrition Info (Per Serving): 341 Calories; 17g Fat; 3.2g Carbs; 42.1g Protein; 0.9g Fiber

Fried Salmon with Asparagus

Servings: 3

Cooking Time: 25 Minute

Ingredients

- 1 cup green asparagus, trimmed
- 2 cloves garlic, sliced
- sea salt and pepper, to taste
- 1 lb salmon fillet, cut into pieces
- 2 tablespoons salted butter
- 2 tablespoons avocado oil
- lemon wedges, optional

Directions:

1. In a medium saucepan, heat the avocado oil. Add the asparagus and garlic. Cook for 5-6 minutes. Season with sea salt and pepper. Set aside.

2. Heat the salted butter in a large skillet. Place the salmon pieces in the skillet.

3. Season with sea salt and pepper. Cook for 4 minutes per side or until cooked through.

4. Serve hot with fresh lemon wedges. Enjoy!

Nutrition Info (Per Serving): 381 Calories; 25g Fat; 4.9g Carbs; 1.3 Fibers; 32.6g Protein

Shrimp Wraps

Servings: 2

Cooking Time: 10 minutes

Ingredients

- 4 oz shrimps
- 2 tbsp coconut flour
- ½ tsp garlic powder
- 1 tbsp avocado oil
- 2 cabbage leaves

Seasoning:
- ¼ tsp salt
- 1/8 tsp ground black pepper
- 1 tbsp water
- 2 tbsp mayonnaise

Directions:

1. Take a shallow dish, place coconut flour in it, and then stir in garlic, powder, salt, and black pepper.
2. Stir in water until smooth and then coat each shrimp in it, one at a time. Take a medium skillet pan, place it over medium heat, add oil and when hot, add shrimps in it and cook for 3 minutes per side until cooked.

3. Distribute shrimps between two cabbage leaves, drizzle with mayonnaise, then roll like a wrap and serve.

Nutrition Info: 265 Calories; 19.9 g Fats; 13.6 g Protein; 3.2 g Net Carb; 3.3 g Fiber

Catfish & Cauliflower Casserole

Servings: 4

Cooking Time: 30 minutes

Ingredients

- 1 tablespoon sesame oil
- 11 ounces cauliflower
- 4 scallions
- 1 garlic clove, minced
- 1 teaspoon fresh ginger root, grated
- Salt and ground black pepper, to taste
- Cayenne pepper, to taste
- 2 sprigs dried thyme, crushed
- 1 sprig rosemary, crushed
- 24 ounces catfish, cut into pieces
- 1/2 cup cream cheese
- 1/2 cup double cream
- 1 egg
- 2 ounces butter, cold

Directions:

1. Start by preheating your oven to 390 degrees F. Now, lightly grease a casserole dish with a nonstick cooking spray.
2. Then, heat the oil in a pan over medium-high heat; once hot, cook the cauliflower and scallions until tender or 5 to

6 minutes. Add the garlic and ginger; continue to sauté 1 minute more.

3. Transfer the vegetables to the prepared casserole dish. Sprinkle with seasonings. Add catfish to the top.

4. In a mixing bowl, thoroughly combine the cream cheese, double cream, and egg. Spread this creamy mixture over the top of your casserole.

5. Top with slices of butter. Bake in the preheated oven for 18 to 22 minutes or until the fish flakes easily with a fork. Bon appétit!

Nutrition Info (Per Serving): 510 Calories; 40g Fat; 5.5g Carbs; 1.6g Fiber; 31.3g Protein

Trout and Endives

Servings: 2

Cooking Time: 15 minutes

Ingredients

- 4 trout fillets
- 2 endives, shredded
- ½ cup shallots, chopped
- 2 tablespoons olive oil
- 1 teaspoon rosemary, dried
- ¼ cup chicken stock
- A pinch of salt and black pepper
- 2 tablespoons chives, chopped

Directions:

1. Heat up a pan with the oil over medium heat, add the shallots and the endives, toss and cook for 2 minutes.

2. Add the fish and cook it for minutes on each side.

3. Add the rest of the ingredients, cook for 8-9 minutes more, divide between plates and serve.

Nutrition Info: calories 200, fat 5, fiber 2, carbs 2, protein 7

Scallops with Broccoli

Servings: 5

Cooking Time: 10 minutes

Ingredients

For Broccoli:

- 1¼ pounds small broccoli florets
- 2 tablespoons unsalted butter, melted

For Scallops:

- 1 tablespoon butter
- 2 garlic cloves, minced
- 1 pound fresh jumbo scallops, side muscles removed
- Salt and ground black pepper, as required
- 2 tablespoons fresh lemon juice
- 2 scallions green part, thinly sliced

Directions:

1. For the broccoli: arrange a steamer basket in a pan of water over medium-high heat and bring to a boil.
2. Place the broccoli in a steamer basket and steam, covered for about 4-5 minutes.
3. Meanwhile, in a large skillet, melt the butter over medium-high heat and sauté the garlic for about 1 minute.

4. Now, add the scallops and cook for about 2 minutes per side.

5. Stir in the salt, black pepper, and lemon juice and remove from heat.

6. Drain the broccoli and transfer it onto a plate.

7. Drizzle the broccoli evenly with melted butter.

8. Divide the cooked broccoli onto serving plates and top with scallops.

9. Garnish with scallions and serve immediately.

Nutrition Info (Per Serving): Calories: 266; Net Carbs: 5.2g; Carbohydrate: 8.3g; Fiber: 3.1g; Protein: 33.1g; Fat: 8.6g; Sugar: 2.2g; Sodium: 430mg

VEGETABLES

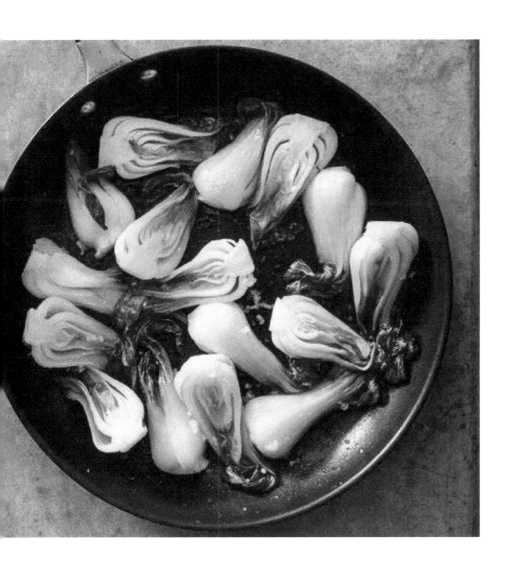

Classic Tangy Ratatouille

Servings: 6

Cooking Time: 47 minutes

Ingredients

- 2 eggplants, chopped
- 3 zucchinis, chopped
- 2 red onions, diced
- 1 (28 oz) can tomatoes
- 2 red bell peppers, cut into chunks
- 1 yellow bell pepper, cut into chunks
- 3 cloves garlic, sliced
- ½ cup basil leaves, chop half
- 4 sprigs thyme
- 1 tbsp balsamic vinegar
- 2 tbsp olive oil
- ½ lemon, zested

Directions:

1. In a casserole pot, heat the olive oil and sauté the eggplants, zucchinis, and bell peppers over medium heat for 5 minutes. Spoon the veggies into a large bowl.

2. In the same pan, sauté garlic, onions, and thyme leaves for 5 minutes and return the cooked veggies to the pan along with the canned tomatoes, balsamic vinegar, chopped basil, salt, and black pepper to taste. Stir and cover the pot, and cook the ingredients on low heat for 30 minutes.

3. Open the lid and stir in the remaining basil leaves, lemon zest, and adjust the seasoning. Turn the heat off. Plate the ratatouille and serve with some low carb crusted bread.

Nutrition Info (Per Serving):

Kcal 154, Fat 12.1g, Net Carbs 5.6g, Protein 1.7g

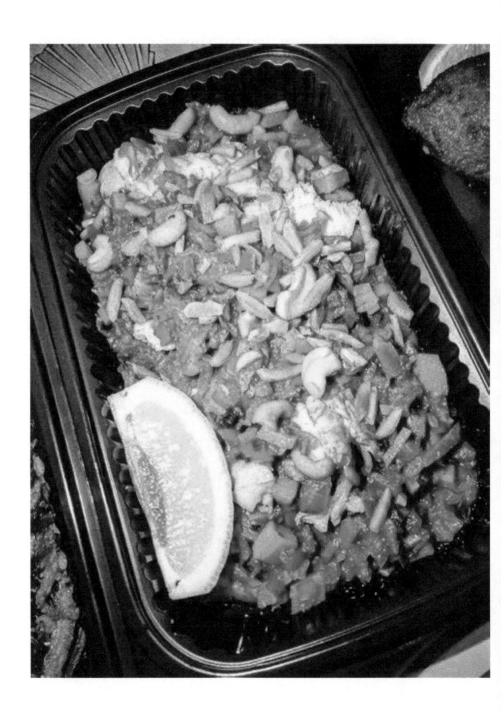

Garlicky Bok Choy

Servings: 4

Cooking Time: 25 minutes

Ingredients

- 2 pounds bok choy, chopped
- 2 tbsp almond oil
- 1 tsp garlic, minced
- ½ tsp thyme
- ½ tsp red pepper flakes, crushed
- Salt and black pepper, to the taste

Directions:

1. Add bok choy in a pot with salted water and cook for minutes over medium heat. Drain and set aside.
2. Place a sauté pan over medium heat and warm oil. Add in garlic and cook until soft. Stir in the bok choy, red pepper, black pepper, salt, and thyme.
3. Add more seasonings if needed and serve with cauli rice.

Nutrition Info (Per Serving): Kcal 118; Fat: 7g, Net Carbs: 13.4g, Protein: 2.9g

Cheesy Zucchini Bake

Servings: 4

Cooking Time: 25 minutes

Ingredients

- 3 large zucchinis, sliced
- 3 tbsp salted butter, melted
- 2 tbsp olive oil
- 1 garlic clove, minced
- 1 tsp dried thyme
- ¼ cup grated mozzarella
- 2/3 cup grated Parmesan

Directions:

1. Preheat oven to 350° F. Pour zucchini in a bowl; add in butter, olive oil, garlic, and thyme; toss to coat. Spread onto a baking dish and sprinkle with the mozzarella and Parmesan cheeses.
2. Bake for minutes or until the cheese melts and is golden.
3. Serve warm with a garden green salad.

Nutrition Info (Per Serving): Cal 194; Net Carbs 3g; Fat 17.2g; Protein 7.4g

Mixed Veggie Salad

Servings: 4

Cooking Time: 20 minutes

Ingredients

For Dressing:

- 1 small avocado, peeled, pitted and chopped
- ¼ cup plain Greek yogurt
- 1 small yellow onion, chopped
- 1 garlic clove, chopped
- 2 tablespoons fresh parsley
- 2 tablespoons fresh lemon juice

For Salad:

- 6 cups fresh spinach, shredded
- 2 medium zucchinis, cut into thin slices
- ½ cup celery, sliced
- ½ cup red bell pepper, seeded and sliced
- ½ cup yellow onion, thinly sliced
- ½ cup cucumber, thinly sliced
- ½ cup cherry tomatoes halved
- ¼ cup Kalamata olives pitted
- ½ cup feta cheese, crumbled

Directions:

1. For the dressing: in a food processor, add all the ingredients and pulse until smooth. For the salad: in a salad bowl, add all the ingredients and mix well.
2. Place the dressing over salad and gently toss to coat well.
3. Serve immediately.

Nutrition Info (Per Serving): Calories: 148; Net Carbs: 6.3g; Carbohydrate: 10.9g; Fiber: 4.6g; Protein: 5.3g; Fat: 10.3g; Sugar: 4.4g; Sodium: 238mg

Broccoli Slaw Salad with Mustard-mayo Dressing

Servings: 6

Cooking Time: 10 minutes

Ingredients

- 2 tbsp granulated swerve
- 1 tbsp Dijon mustard
- 1 tbsp olive oil
- 4 cups broccoli slaw
- ⅓ cup mayonnaise, sugar-free
- 1 tsp celery seeds
- 1 ½ tbsp apple cider vinegar
- Salt and black pepper, to taste

Directions:

1. Whisk together the ingredients except for the broccoli slaw. Place broccoli slaw in a large salad bowl. Pour the dressing over. Mix with your hands to combine well.

Nutrition Info (Per Serving): Kcal 110, Fat: 10g, Net Carbs: 2g, Protein: 3g

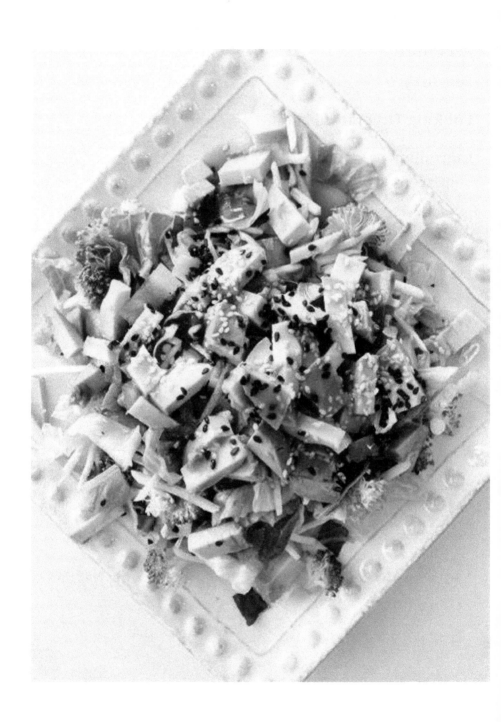

DESSERT

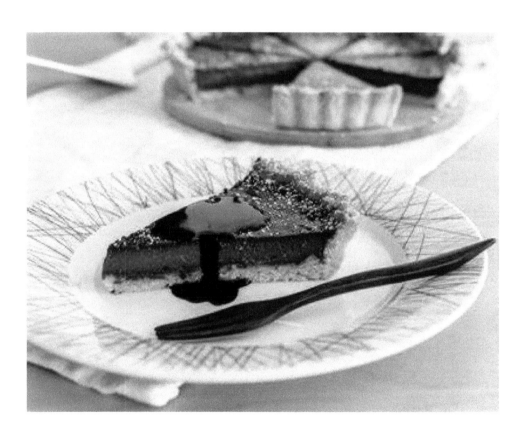

Simple Chocolate Tart

Servings: 4

Cooking Time: 25 minutes

Ingredients

For the crust:

- 1 1/3 cups almond flour
- 1 ½ tsp coconut flour
- ¼ cup swerve sugar
- 1 ½ tsp cold water
- 3 tbsp cold butter

For the filling:

- 4 oz heavy cream
- 4 oz dark chocolate chips
- 1/3 cup erythritol

Directions:

1. Preheat oven to 350° F. In a food processor, blend almond and coconut flours, swerve, water, and butter until smooth. Spread the dough in a greased round baking pan and bake for minutes; let cool.

2. For the filling, heat heavy cream and chocolate chips in a pot over medium heat until chocolate melts; whisk in erythritol.

3. Pour the filling into the crust, gently tap on a flat surface to release air bubbles and chill for 1 hour.

4. Remove from the fridge, and serve.

Nutrition Info (Per Serving): Cal 177; Net Carbs 1g; Fat 19g; Protein 3g

Chocolate Chip Blondies

Servings: 2

Cooking Time: 30 minutes

Ingredients

- 1/2 cup almond flour
- 1/4 teaspoon cream of tartar
- 1/4 teaspoon baking soda
- A pinch of salt
- A pinch of grated nutmeg
- 1 egg, whisked
- 1/4 cup butter, melted
- 1 tablespoon milk
- 1/2 cup Swerve sweetener
- 1/2 teaspoon vanilla bean seeds
- 1/4 cup chocolate chips, unsweetened

Directions:

1. In a mixing bowl, thoroughly combine the almond flour, cream of tartar, baking soda, salt, and nutmeg. In another bowl, whisk the egg, butter, milk, and sweetener.

2. Add the almond flour mixture to the egg mixture and mix to combine well. Afterwards, stir in the vanilla bean seeds and chocolate chips; stir again using a spatula.

100

3. Scrape the batter into a parchment-lined baking pan. Bake in the preheated oven at 0 degrees F for 22 to 25 minutes. Don't over-bake; the blondies should remain juicy in the center.

4. Let it cool down; then, cut into equal size squares and enjoy!

Nutrition Info (Per Serving): 347 Calories; 34g Fat; 5.2g Total Carbs; 5.7g Protein; 2.8g Fiber

Strawberry Stew

Servings: 4

Cooking Time: 15 minutes

Ingredients

- ½ cup swerve
- 1 pound strawberries, halved
- 2 cups of water
- 1 teaspoon vanilla extract

Directions:

1. In a pan, combine the strawberries with the swerve and the other ingredients, toss gently, bring to a simmer and cook over medium heat for minutes.
2. Divide into bowls and serve cold.

Nutrition Info: calories 40, fat 4.3, fiber 2.3, carbs 3.4, protein 0.8

Passion Fruit Cheesecake Slices

Servings: 8

Cooking Time: 15 minutes + Cooling Time

Ingredients

- 1 cup crushed almond biscuits
- ½ cup melted butter Filling:
- 1 ½ cups cream cheese
- ¾ cup swerve sugar
- 1 ½ whipping cream
- 1 tsp vanilla bean paste
- 4-6 tbsp cold water
- 1 tbsp gelatin powder

Passionfruit jelly:
- 1 cup passion fruit pulp
- ¼ cup swerve confectioner's sugar
- 1 tsp gelatin powder
- ¼ cup water, room temperature

Directions:

1. Mix the crushed biscuits and butter in a bowl, spoon into a spring-form pan, and use the spoon's back to level at the bottom. Set aside in the fridge. Put the cream cheese,

swerve sugar, and vanilla paste into a bowl, and use the hand mixer to whisk until smooth; set aside.

2. In a bowl, add tbsp of cold water and sprinkle 1 tbsp of gelatin powder. Let dissolve for 5 minutes. Pour the gelatin liquid along with the whipping cream in the cheese mixture and fold gently.

3. Remove the spring-form pan from the refrigerator and pour over the mixture. Return to the fridge.

4. For the passionfruit jelly: add 2 tbsp of cold water and sprinkle 1 tsp of gelatin powder. Let dissolve for 5 minutes. Pour the confectioner's sugar and ¼ cup of water into it.

5. Mix and stir in passion fruit pulp.

6. Remove the cake again and pour the jelly over it. Swirl the pan to make the jelly level up. Place the pan back into the fridge to cool for 2 hours. When completely set, remove and unlock the spring-pan. Lift the pan from the cake and slice the dessert.

Nutrition Info (Per Serving): Kcal 287, Fat 18g, Net Carbs 6.1g, Protein 4.4g

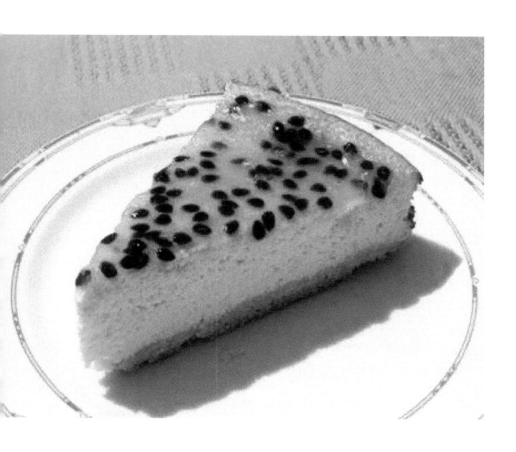

Lemon Mug Cake

Preparation Time: 5 minutes

Cooking Time: 2 minutes

Servings: 1

Ingredients:

- 1 egg, lightly beaten
- 1/2 tsp. lemon rind
- 1 tbsp. butter, melted
- 1 1/2 tbsp. fresh lemon juice
- 2 tbsp. erythritol
- 1/4 tsp. baking powder, gluten-free
- 1/4 cup almond flour

Directions:

1. In a bowl or container, mix almond flour, baking powder, and sweetener.
2. Add egg, lemon juice, and melted butter in almond flour mixture and whisk until well combined.
3. Pour cake mixture into the microwave-safe mug and microwave for 90 seconds.
4. Serve and enjoy.

Nutrition: Calories: 275 Fats: 5.9g Fiber: 2.4g Carbohydrates: 1.3 g Protein: 4.1g

Strawberry Mousse

Preparation Time: 10 minutes

Cooking Time: 5 minutes

Servings: 2

Ingredients:

- 1 cup heavy whipping cream
- 1 cup fresh strawberries, chopped
- 2 tbsp. Swerve
- 1 cup cream cheese

Directions:

1. Add heavy whipping cream in a bowl and beat until thickened using a hand mixer.
2. Add sweetener and cream cheese and beat well. Add strawberries and fold well.
3. Pour in serving glasses and place in the refrigerator for 1-2 hours. Serve chilled and enjoy.

Nutrition:

Calories: 219 Fat: 8g Fiber: 3.1g Carbohydrates: 1.9 g Protein: 1.2g

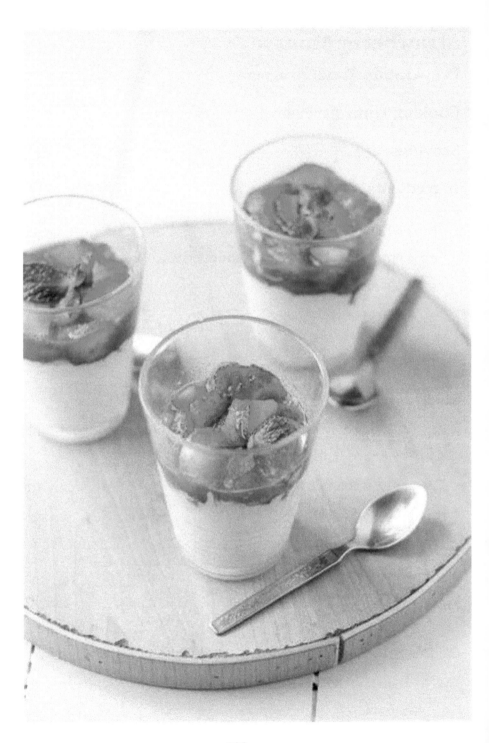

Lightning Source UK Ltd.
Milton Keynes UK
UKHW020758230621
386009UK00001B/14